Copyrighted material

SEXUAL

POWER

DIET

Copyrighted material

Copyright © 2024 by Francesco Rosato

All rights reserved. No part of this book may be reproduced or transmitted in any form or by any means, electronic or mechanical, including photocopying, recording, or by any information storage and retrieval system, without permission in writing from the author, except for brief quotations in reviews and other non-commercial uses permitted by copyright law.

The information contained in this book is for educational purposes only. The author and publisher make no representations or warranties with respect to the accuracy or completeness of the contents of this book and specifically disclaim any implied warranties of merchantability or fitness for a particular purpose. The advice and strategies contained herein may not be suitable for every situation. The author and publisher shall not be liable for any loss of profit or any other commercial damages, including but not limited to special, incidental, consequential, or other damages.

Copyrighted material

About the author: Francesco Rosato is a renowned Personal Trainer, sports entrepreneur, and author specializing in maximizing sexual vitality and wellness. As a devoted Personal Trainer, Francesco is deeply passionate about guiding individuals to achieve their peak sexual fitness and wellness. Through innovative approaches tailored specifically to enhancing sexual performance, Francesco has gained recognition as a trusted mentor and motivator in the realm of sexual health.

Beyond his contributions as a fitness professional, Francesco is a successful entrepreneur in the sexual wellness industry, possessing a profound understanding of the crucial role mental resilience and determination play in attaining sexual fulfillment. Drawing from his personal experiences and professional acumen, Francesco is committed to aiding individuals in overcoming obstacles to their sexual vitality, enabling them to lead more gratifying lives.

Francesco's bestselling motivational works have impacted countless readers, inspiring them to transcend limitations and embrace a life of heightened sexual prowess, satisfaction, and purpose. Through his writing, Francesco shares practical strategies, heartfelt encouragement, and empowering narratives of transformation, equipping readers with the tools and inspiration necessary to embark on their own journey toward unleashing their sexual potential.

Copyrighted material

With his distinctive amalgamation of personal insight, professional proficiency, and unwavering dedication to empowering others, Francesco Rosato stands as a leading advocate in the domain of sexual health and wellness, inspiring individuals worldwide to harness their innate sexual power and live vibrantly fulfilling lives.

Copyrighted material

Contents

Introduction 7

Chapter 1: Fundamentals of Sexual Health...................... 12

Definition of Sexual Health 12

Connection between Diet and Sexual Health 14

Chapter 2: Nutrition and Sexual Hormones...................... 18

Role of Sexual Hormones in Health and Well-being 18

Foods That Influence the Production of Sexual Hormones20

Impact of Hormones on Libido and Sexual Function 23

Chapter 3: Aphrodisiac Foods 26

Aphrodisiacs: A Detailed Exploration of Their History and Effects 26

Foods Known to Enhance Libido and Sexual Function 29

Recipes and tips for incorporating aphrodisiacs into daily diet 35

Chapter 4: Nutrition for Fertility 69

Importance of diet for fertility...................................... 69

Foods that promote reproductive health 72

Advice for couples trying to conceive 75

Chapter 5: Diet and Sexual Dysfunctions........................... 79

Negative effects of poor diet on sexual dysfunctions........ 79

Foods that may worsen sexual dysfunctions 81

Dietary advice for addressing sexual dysfunctions............ 84

Copyrighted material

Chapter 6: Dietary Program to Enhance Sexual Health 88

Practical guide for a diet aimed at sexual health...............88

Meal preparation tips 91

Strategies for maintaining a healthy diet long-term 93

Chapter 7: Supplements and Natural Remedies 97

Dietary supplements useful for improving sexual health. .97

Natural remedies and herbs that can support sexual function 100

Considerations regarding the safety and efficacy of supplements and remedies...103

Conclusion 107

Free Gift 111

Copyrighted material

Introduction

In the ever-evolving landscape of health and wellness, the interplay between nutrition and various facets of well-being has garnered increasing attention. From physical fitness to mental resilience, the foods we consume exert a profound influence on our overall vitality and quality of life. Yet, amidst discussions on diet and health, one crucial aspect often remains obscured: the intricate relationship between dietary choices and sexual health.

Sexual health represents a holistic continuum encompassing physical, emotional, and social dimensions, as recognized by leading health organizations worldwide, including the World Health Organization (WHO). It transcends mere absence of disease or dysfunction, embodying a state of complete well-being and fulfillment in relation to sexuality and intimate relationships. Despite its paramount importance, sexual health remains an underexplored terrain in mainstream discourse, particularly concerning the pivotal role of nutrition in shaping sexual function and satisfaction.

The foundation of sexual vitality lies in the intricate orchestration of physiological processes, hormonal

Copyrighted material

balance, and psychological well-being. Within this complex framework, diet emerges as a potent modulator, capable of influencing myriad factors crucial to sexual health. From the regulation of sex hormones to the promotion of cardiovascular health and the modulation of neurotransmitter activity, the foods we consume wield profound effects on our sexual vitality and prowess.

The journey toward optimal sexual health begins with a comprehensive understanding of the interplay between diet and sexual function. In this introductory chapter, we embark on an immersive exploration of the multifaceted relationship between nutrition and sexual health. Through an integrative lens that merges scientific inquiry with experiential wisdom, we unravel the nuances of how dietary choices shape libido, arousal, reproductive function, and overall sexual satisfaction.

Our odyssey traverses the vast landscape of nutritional science, delving into the intricate biochemistry underpinning sexual health and exploring the role of specific nutrients, phytochemicals, and dietary patterns in fostering sexual vitality. We dissect the aphrodisiac properties of select foods, dissecting their mechanisms of action and unveiling culinary delights that tantalize the senses while kindling the flames of desire.

Moreover, we probe beyond the realm of individual nutrients, venturing into the realm of dietary patterns and lifestyle factors that underpin sexual well-being.

Copyrighted material

From the Mediterranean diet's renowned cardiovascular benefits to the therapeutic potential of plant-based nutrition in ameliorating sexual dysfunctions, we navigate a rich tapestry of dietary strategies aimed at nurturing sexual vitality and resilience.

Yet, our exploration extends beyond the physiological realm, encompassing the intricate interplay between diet, psychology, and relational dynamics in shaping sexual satisfaction and intimacy. Through insightful anecdotes, evidence-based strategies, and practical recommendations, we illuminate pathways toward fostering open communication, deepening emotional intimacy, and cultivating a shared culinary journey that enhances not only physical pleasure but also emotional connection and relational fulfillment.

Join us on this transformative odyssey as we navigate the nexus of nutrition and sexuality, charting a course toward enhanced sexual vitality, enriched intimacy, and empowered well-being. Through the prism of the Sexual Power Diet, we embark on a journey of self-discovery, nourishing not only our bodies but also our spirits, and forging deeper connections within ourselves and with our beloved partners.

Objectives of the Book:

1. Educate: Unlock the Secrets to Sexual Vitality: Dive into the fascinating world of "Sexual Power Diet" and discover

Copyrighted material

how the foods you eat impact every aspect of your sexual health. From boosting libido to enhancing satisfaction, this book is your comprehensive guide to harnessing the power of nutrition for a vibrant and fulfilling sex life.

2. Illuminate: Shedding Light on the Science of Sex: Embark on a journey of discovery as we delve deep into the science behind nutrition and sexual function. Through cutting-edge research, expert insights, and real-life stories, "Sexual Power Diet" illuminates the complex interplay between diet and sexual vitality, empowering you with knowledge to transform your intimate experiences.

3. Empower: Take Control of Your Sexual Well-Being: Say goodbye to guesswork and confusion with actionable strategies and practical recommendations tailored to your lifestyle. Whether you're seeking to reignite passion, improve performance, or enhance fertility, "Sexual Power Diet" equips you with the tools and confidence to make informed choices that nourish your sexual health from within.

4. Destigmatize: Breaking Barriers, Opening Minds: It's time to challenge outdated beliefs and break free from societal taboos surrounding sexuality and nutrition. With candid conversations, myth-busting facts, and a compassionate approach, "Sexual Power Diet" creates a safe space for open dialogue, allowing you to explore your sexual well-being with confidence and clarity.

Copyrighted material

5. Inspire: Ignite Your Passion, Embrace Your Potential: Get ready to embark on a transformative journey toward holistic well-being and self-discovery. By embracing the principles of the Sexual Power Diet, you'll not only revitalize your body but also nurture deeper connections with yourself and your partner, paving the way for a life filled with vitality, intimacy, and unparalleled satisfaction.

Copyrighted material

Chapter 1: Fundamentals of Sexual Health

Definition of Sexual Health

Sexual health is a multifaceted and dynamic aspect of overall well-being that encompasses physical, emotional, mental, and social dimensions of human sexuality. It represents a state of holistic harmony and vitality in relation to one's sexual identity, experiences, and relationships. At its essence, sexual health is not merely the absence of disease or dysfunction but rather the presence of positive and affirming attitudes, behaviors, and experiences related to sexuality.

Physical Dimension:

From a physical standpoint, sexual health encompasses a range of factors that contribute to the well-being of sexual organs and bodily functions. This includes aspects such as reproductive health, sexual function, and the prevention and management of sexually transmitted infections (STIs) and other sexual health conditions. It also extends to the promotion of sexual pleasure, vitality, and satisfaction through healthy lifestyle choices, including diet, exercise, and regular healthcare.

Emotional Dimension:

Emotional well-being is intricately linked to sexual health, encompassing feelings of self-esteem, confidence, and

Copyrighted material

emotional intimacy within sexual relationships. It involves a sense of comfort and acceptance with one's own body and desires, as well as the ability to communicate openly and authentically with sexual partners. Emotional resilience and coping mechanisms also play a crucial role in navigating the complexities of sexual experiences and relationships.

Mental Dimension:

The mental aspect of sexual health encompasses cognitive processes, attitudes, and beliefs related to sexuality. This includes the development of accurate sexual knowledge and understanding, as well as the cultivation of healthy sexual attitudes and values. Mental health disorders, such as anxiety, depression, and trauma, can significantly impact sexual well-being and may require specialized support and intervention to address.

Social Dimension:

Social factors, including cultural norms, societal attitudes, and interpersonal relationships, profoundly influence sexual health outcomes. This dimension of sexual health encompasses the ability to form and maintain healthy, respectful, and consensual sexual relationships, as well as the negotiation of sexual boundaries and preferences within a social context. It also involves addressing issues

Copyrighted material

of gender inequality, discrimination, and violence that may impact sexual well-being.

Promotion of Sexual Rights and Responsibilities:

Central to the concept of sexual health is the recognition and promotion of sexual rights and responsibilities. This includes the right to accurate sexual information, comprehensive sexual education, and access to sexual and reproductive healthcare services. It also entails the responsibility to respect and uphold the sexual rights of others, including the right to autonomy, privacy, and bodily integrity.

In summary, sexual health is a multifaceted and dynamic construct that encompasses physical, emotional, mental, and social dimensions of well-being. It is characterized by a positive and affirming approach to sexuality, rooted in respect, autonomy, and consent. By addressing the diverse needs and experiences of individuals, promoting sexual rights and responsibilities, and fostering an inclusive and supportive environment, we can strive to achieve optimal sexual health for all.

Connection between Diet and Sexual Health

The relationship between diet and sexual health is multifaceted, encompassing a variety of physiological, psychological, and emotional factors that influence sexual function, desire, and satisfaction. Here, we explore the intricate connections between dietary habits and sexual well-being in greater detail:

Copyrighted material

1. Nutrient Intake and Hormonal Balance: Nutrients play a vital role in the regulation of sex hormones, which are essential for sexual function and libido. For example, zinc is crucial for testosterone production in men, while vitamin D has been linked to testosterone levels in both men and women. Additionally, certain amino acids, such as arginine and carnitine, are involved in nitric oxide synthesis, which helps regulate blood flow to the genitals and is essential for achieving and maintaining erections.

2. Cardiovascular Health and Blood Flow: A healthy cardiovascular system is paramount for sexual health, as adequate blood flow is necessary for arousal and erectile function. Diets rich in fruits, vegetables, whole grains, and lean proteins promote cardiovascular health by lowering blood pressure, reducing inflammation, and improving endothelial function, all of which contribute to enhanced blood flow to the genitals. Conversely, diets high in saturated fats, trans fats, and refined sugars can lead to cardiovascular disease, atherosclerosis, and impaired blood flow, negatively impacting sexual function.

3. Body Weight and Body Composition: Maintaining a healthy body weight and body composition is essential for sexual health and satisfaction. Obesity and excess body fat have been associated with various sexual dysfunctions, including erectile dysfunction, reduced libido, and infertility. Excess adipose tissue can lead to hormonal imbalances, such as elevated estrogen levels in men, which can impair sexual function. Moreover, obesity is linked to psychological factors, such as body image issues and low self-esteem, which can further exacerbate sexual problems.

Copyrighted material

4. Psychological and Emotional Well-being: Dietary habits can significantly influence psychological and emotional well-being, which in turn impact sexual health. For example, diets rich in omega-3 fatty acids, found in fatty fish, walnuts, and flaxseeds, have been associated with improved mood and reduced symptoms of depression and anxiety. Conversely, diets high in processed foods, refined sugars, and unhealthy fats can lead to mood swings, fatigue, and irritability, which can negatively affect sexual desire and satisfaction.

5. Energy Levels and Fatigue: Energy levels and fatigue play a crucial role in sexual arousal and performance. Diets that provide sustained energy through a balance of carbohydrates, proteins, and healthy fats can support optimal energy levels and reduce fatigue, enhancing sexual vitality and endurance. On the other hand, diets high in simple sugars and refined carbohydrates can lead to energy crashes and fatigue, impairing sexual function and enjoyment.

6. Micronutrients and Sexual Health: In addition to macronutrients, micronutrients such as vitamins and minerals also play a vital role in sexual health. For example, vitamin C, vitamin E, and antioxidants help protect against oxidative stress, which can damage sperm cells and impair fertility. Similarly, folate, zinc, and selenium are essential for sperm production and motility. Deficiencies in these micronutrients can negatively impact reproductive health and fertility.

7. Gut Health and Sexual Well-being: Emerging research suggests a link between gut health and sexual well-being. The gut microbiota, composed of trillions of microorganisms, plays a crucial role in immune function, metabolism, and hormonal

Copyrighted material

regulation. Imbalances in gut bacteria, known as dysbiosis, have been associated with various health conditions, including obesity, diabetes, and inflammation, which can impact sexual health. Diets high in fiber, prebiotics, and probiotics support a healthy gut microbiota, potentially improving sexual function and overall well-being.

In summary, the connection between diet and sexual health is multifaceted, with dietary habits influencing various physiological, psychological, and emotional factors that contribute to sexual well-being. By adopting a balanced and nutritious diet that supports hormonal balance, cardiovascular health, positive body image, psychological well-being, and sustained energy levels, individuals can enhance their sexual health and enjoy a more fulfilling and satisfying sex life.

Copyrighted material

Chapter 2: Nutrition and Sexual Hormones

Role of Sexual Hormones in Health and Well-being

Sexual hormones, including testosterone, estrogen, and progesterone, play a crucial role in maintaining overall health and well-being, with their effects extending beyond reproductive function to influence various physiological processes throughout the body. These hormones are essential for the development and functioning of reproductive organs, as well as for regulating numerous bodily functions, including metabolism, bone health, mood regulation, and cardiovascular health.

1. Testosterone:

Testosterone is the primary male sex hormone, although it is also present in smaller quantities in females. In men, testosterone plays a key role in the development of male reproductive organs, such as the testes and prostate gland, as well as in the production of sperm. Beyond its reproductive functions, testosterone also influences muscle mass, bone density, fat distribution, and red blood cell production. In women, testosterone contributes to sexual arousal, libido, and overall well-being.

2. Estrogen:

Copyrighted material

Estrogen is the primary female sex hormone, although it is also present in men in smaller amounts. In women, estrogen is responsible for the development of female reproductive organs, such as the ovaries, uterus, and breasts, as well as for regulating the menstrual cycle and supporting pregnancy. Estrogen also plays a role in bone health, cardiovascular health, mood regulation, and cognitive function. In men, estrogen helps regulate libido, erectile function, and bone density.

3. Progesterone:

Progesterone is a hormone produced primarily in the ovaries in women and in smaller amounts in the adrenal glands in both men and women. In women, progesterone plays a crucial role in regulating the menstrual cycle, supporting pregnancy, and preparing the uterus for implantation of a fertilized egg. Progesterone also influences mood, sleep, and immune function. In men, progesterone is involved in the production of testosterone and supports overall reproductive health.

Effects of Hormonal Imbalance:

Imbalances in sexual hormones can have significant effects on health and well-being, leading to a range of symptoms and health issues. For example, low testosterone levels in men may contribute to decreased libido, erectile dysfunction, fatigue, muscle loss, and mood changes. In women, hormonal imbalances, such as

Copyrighted material

low estrogen or progesterone levels, can lead to irregular menstrual cycles, hot flashes, mood swings, and decreased libido.

Nutrition and Hormonal Balance:

Diet plays a crucial role in supporting hormonal balance, as certain nutrients are essential for hormone production and regulation. For example, adequate intake of zinc, magnesium, and vitamin D is important for testosterone production, while phytoestrogens found in foods like soy may help support estrogen levels in women. A balanced diet rich in fruits, vegetables, whole grains, lean proteins, and healthy fats provides the nutrients necessary for optimal hormonal function.

In conclusion, sexual hormones play a vital role in maintaining overall health and well-being, influencing various physiological processes throughout the body. By understanding the role of sexual hormones and adopting a balanced diet that supports hormonal balance, individuals can promote optimal health and vitality.

Foods That Influence the Production of Sexual Hormones

The production and regulation of sexual hormones, including testosterone, estrogen, and progesterone, are influenced by a variety of factors, including genetics, age, lifestyle, and dietary habits. While dietary choices alone may not drastically alter hormone levels, certain

Copyrighted material

nutrients found in foods can support hormonal balance and optimize reproductive health. Here are some key nutrients and foods that may influence the production of sexual hormones:

1. Zinc: Zinc is an essential mineral that plays a critical role in hormone production, including testosterone and estrogen. Foods rich in zinc include oysters, beef, poultry, seafood, pumpkin seeds, nuts, and legumes. Incorporating these zinc-rich foods into your diet can help support healthy hormone levels.

2. Magnesium: Magnesium is another important mineral involved in hormone regulation and production. It helps to support adrenal function, which is important for the synthesis of sex hormones. Foods high in magnesium include leafy green vegetables, nuts, seeds, whole grains, and legumes.

3. Vitamin D: Vitamin D is crucial for overall health, including hormonal balance. It has been shown to play a role in testosterone production and regulation. Foods rich in vitamin D include fatty fish (such as salmon and mackerel), egg yolks, fortified dairy and plant-based milk, and mushrooms exposed to sunlight.

4. Omega-3 Fatty Acids: Omega-3 fatty acids are essential fats that play a role in hormone production and inflammation regulation. They are found in fatty fish (such as salmon, mackerel, and sardines), flaxseeds, chia

Copyrighted material

seeds, walnuts, and hemp seeds. Incorporating omega-3-rich foods into your diet may help support hormonal balance.

5. Phytoestrogens: Phytoestrogens are plant compounds that mimic the effects of estrogen in the body. While they are not identical to human estrogen, they can bind to estrogen receptors and exert weak estrogenic effects. Foods rich in phytoestrogens include soy products (such as tofu, tempeh, and edamame), flaxseeds, sesame seeds, and legumes.

6. Vitamin B6: Vitamin B6 is involved in the synthesis of neurotransmitters and steroid hormones, including sex hormones like estrogen and progesterone. Foods rich in vitamin B6 include poultry, fish, bananas, potatoes, avocados, nuts, and seeds.

7. Antioxidants: Antioxidants, such as vitamin C, vitamin E, and selenium, help protect cells from oxidative stress and may support overall hormonal balance. Foods rich in antioxidants include fruits (such as berries, citrus fruits, and kiwi), vegetables (such as spinach, kale, and bell peppers), nuts, seeds, and whole grains.

8. Healthy Fats: Healthy fats, such as monounsaturated and polyunsaturated fats, are important for hormone production and regulation. They are found in foods like avocados, olive oil, nuts, seeds, and fatty fish.

Copyrighted material

While these foods can support overall hormonal balance when included as part of a balanced diet, it's important to remember that individual hormone levels are influenced by a variety of factors. Additionally, consulting with a healthcare professional or registered dietitian can provide personalized recommendations for optimizing hormonal health through diet.

Impact of Hormones on Libido and Sexual Function

Hormones play a crucial role in regulating libido and sexual function, influencing a complex array of physiological processes that contribute to sexual arousal, performance, and satisfaction. Testosterone, estrogen, progesterone, and other hormones engage in an intricate dance within the body, modulating sexual desire, arousal, and response to sexual stimuli.

Testosterone, known as the quintessential male hormone but also present in females in lesser quantities, is critical for libido in both sexes. In males, it is essential for the development of male sexual characteristics and for maintaining libido and sexual function. Low testosterone levels can lead to reduced libido and erectile dysfunction. In females, testosterone contributes to libido and sexual arousal, and fluctuations in its levels during the menstrual cycle can influence libido.

Estrogens, primary female hormones, affect desire, arousal, and sexual lubrication in women. Fluctuations in estrogen levels during the menstrual cycle can impact

Copyrighted material

libido, with higher levels associated with increased sexual desire. During menopause, when estrogen levels decline, some women may experience decreased libido and sexual function.

Progesterone, primarily produced in women's ovaries and in smaller amounts in both men's and women's adrenal glands, influences sexual function. Although primarily known for its role in regulating the menstrual cycle and supporting pregnancy, progesterone may affect libido, with high levels relative to estrogen potentially reducing its intensity.

Prolactin, a hormone produced by the pituitary gland, increases after orgasm, causing a temporary decrease in libido, known as the refractory period, in both men and women. Elevated prolactin levels may be associated with reduced libido and sexual function, especially in men.

Oxytocin, known as the "love hormone," is involved in social bonding, intimacy, and sexual arousal. It increases during sexual activity, contributing to feelings of pleasure and emotional connection. Oxytocin also plays a role in uterine contractions during orgasm and may influence vaginal lubrication and orgasm intensity.

Cortisol, produced by the adrenal glands in response to stress, can influence libido and sexual function. Chronic stress and elevated cortisol levels can disrupt hormonal

Copyrighted material

balance and affect mood, energy levels, and overall well-being, with negative consequences for sexual health.

In conclusion, hormones play a fundamental role in regulating libido and sexual function, with fluctuations in their levels influencing desire, arousal, and sexual satisfaction in both sexes. Maintaining hormonal balance through healthy lifestyle choices, stress management, and medical interventions when necessary is essential for promoting optimal sexual health and overall well-being.

Copyrighted material

Chapter 3: Aphrodisiac Foods

Aphrodisiacs: A Detailed Exploration of Their History and Effects

Ancient Origins:

The fascination with aphrodisiacs dates back to ancient civilizations, where various cultures and societies explored the use of substances to enhance sexual desire and performance. In ancient Egypt, for example, foods like honey and figs were revered for their purported aphrodisiac properties and were offered to fertility deities in hopes of increasing virility and fertility. Similarly, in ancient Greece, foods like almonds and olives were believed to stimulate desire and were incorporated into romantic rituals and celebrations.

Historical References:

References to aphrodisiacs can also be found in classical literature and mythology. In Greek mythology, Aphrodite, the goddess of love, was often associated with certain foods and substances believed to enhance passion and desire. The Kama Sutra, an ancient Indian text on sexuality and relationships, contains references to various aphrodisiacs and their effects on sexual pleasure and satisfaction.

Cultural Practices:

Copyrighted material

The use of aphrodisiacs is often deeply rooted in cultural practices and traditions surrounding sexuality and fertility. In many indigenous cultures, rituals involving the consumption of specific herbs, roots, or animal parts are believed to enhance libido and sexual potency. For example, in some African cultures, the consumption of animal testicles or certain herbs is believed to increase sexual stamina and vigor.

Natural Aphrodisiacs:

Throughout history, numerous natural substances have been hailed as aphrodisiacs due to their perceived effects on sexual desire and arousal. These include:

- Ginseng: Used in traditional Chinese medicine for centuries, ginseng is believed to improve libido and sexual performance by increasing blood flow and reducing stress.

- Maca Root: Native to the Andes Mountains, maca root is renowned for its purported aphrodisiac properties and is believed to enhance libido and fertility.

- Damiana: Native to Central and South America, damiana is a shrub traditionally used as an aphrodisiac and is believed to increase sexual desire and pleasure.

Copyrighted material

- Oysters: Oysters have long been associated with aphrodisiac effects due to their high zinc content, which is essential for testosterone production and sexual health.

- Chocolate: Chocolate contains compounds such as phenylethylamine and serotonin, which are believed to promote feelings of pleasure and arousal.

Scientific Perspectives:

While the efficacy of aphrodisiacs is often debated, modern scientific research has shed light on the potential mechanisms underlying their effects on sexual desire and function. Some substances, such as ginseng and maca root, have been studied for their potential aphrodisiac effects, with some evidence suggesting improvements in libido and sexual performance. However, more research is needed to fully understand the mechanisms and efficacy of these substances.

Cultural Significance:

Despite the scientific debate surrounding their efficacy, aphrodisiacs continue to hold cultural significance in many societies. Whether used in traditional rituals and ceremonies or embraced as exotic delicacies, aphrodisiacs remain a symbol of sensuality, romance, and the pursuit of enhanced sexual experiences.

Copyrighted material

Conclusion:

The history of aphrodisiacs is rich and multifaceted, spanning cultures and civilizations throughout the ages. From ancient rituals and traditions to modern scientific research, the fascination with substances that enhance sexual desire and pleasure continues to captivate human curiosity and imagination. Whether rooted in mythology, folklore, or scientific inquiry, the allure of aphrodisiacs persists as a testament to the enduring human quest for passion, intimacy, and sexual fulfillment.

Foods Known to Enhance Libido and Sexual Function

The relationship between diet and sexual health is well-established, with certain foods known for their potential to enhance libido, arousal, and sexual function. Incorporating these foods into your diet can provide essential nutrients and compounds that support overall sexual well-being. Here are some foods known for their aphrodisiac properties:

1. Oysters: Oysters have long been celebrated as a natural aphrodisiac due to their high zinc content, which is essential for testosterone production and maintaining healthy sperm levels. Additionally, oysters contain amino acids that are believed to increase the production of sex hormones.

2. Dark Chocolate: Dark chocolate contains flavonoids, which are antioxidants that have been associated with

Copyrighted material

increased blood flow and improved cardiovascular health. Chocolate also contains phenylethylamine, a compound that stimulates the release of endorphins, promoting feelings of pleasure and arousal.

3. Watermelon: Watermelon contains citrulline, an amino acid that relaxes blood vessels and may improve blood flow, similar to the effects of Viagra. This can lead to enhanced arousal and improved erectile function.

4. Ginseng: Ginseng has been used for centuries in traditional medicine to enhance libido and sexual performance. It is believed to improve blood circulation and increase energy levels, leading to improved sexual function.

5. Maca Root: Maca root, native to the Andes Mountains, is known for its potential to increase libido and improve sexual function. It is believed to balance hormones and increase energy levels, supporting overall sexual vitality.

6. Avocado: Avocado is rich in vitamin E, which is essential for hormone production and may promote blood flow, leading to increased arousal and sexual satisfaction. Additionally, avocados contain healthy fats that support heart health, which is important for overall sexual function.

7. Almonds: Almonds are a good source of zinc, selenium, and vitamin E, all of which are important for reproductive health and hormone production. Additionally, almonds

Copyrighted material

contain arginine, an amino acid that has been shown to improve blood flow and erectile function.

8. Chili Peppers: Chili peppers contain capsaicin, a compound that stimulates nerve endings and increases heart rate, leading to feelings of arousal. Additionally, capsaicin may release endorphins, promoting feelings of pleasure and well-being.

9. Strawberries: Strawberries are rich in vitamin C and antioxidants, which support cardiovascular health and improve blood flow. They also contain compounds that may enhance libido and sexual pleasure.

10. Asparagus: Asparagus is rich in folate, which is essential for the production of histamine, a neurotransmitter involved in sexual arousal. Additionally, asparagus contains vitamin E, which supports hormone production and may enhance sexual function.

11. Bananas: Bananas are rich in potassium and vitamin B6, which are important for hormone production and energy levels. They also contain bromelain, an enzyme that may help increase libido and improve sexual function.

12. Figs: Figs are considered a symbol of fertility and have been associated with aphrodisiac properties since ancient times. They are rich in vitamins, minerals, and antioxidants that support overall health and may enhance sexual desire and arousal.

Copyrighted material

13.	Pomegranates: Pomegranates are rich in antioxidants, particularly polyphenols, which support cardiovascular health and improve blood flow. Some studies suggest that pomegranate juice may improve erectile function and enhance sexual satisfaction.

14. Honey: Honey has been used as a natural sweetener and remedy for various ailments for centuries. It contains boron, a mineral that may help regulate hormone levels, as well as antioxidants that support overall health. Honey is also associated with increased energy levels and may enhance sexual desire.

15. Ginseng Tea: In addition to ginseng root, ginseng tea is another popular form of consumption. Ginseng tea is believed to have similar aphrodisiac effects as ginseng root, promoting increased libido and sexual vitality.

16. Pumpkin Seeds: Pumpkin seeds are rich in zinc, which is essential for testosterone production and sperm health. They also contain omega-3 fatty acids and antioxidants that support cardiovascular health and may enhance sexual function.

17.	Celery: Celery contains androstenone and androstenol, pheromones that are believed to increase sexual attraction and arousal. Additionally, celery is rich in vitamins, minerals, and antioxidants that support overall health and may contribute to enhanced sexual function.

Copyrighted material

18. Cinnamon: Cinnamon is a spice that has been used for centuries for its aromatic and medicinal properties. Some studies suggest that cinnamon may improve blood flow and circulation, which could enhance sexual function and arousal.

19. Saffron: Saffron is one of the most expensive spices in the world and has been prized for its culinary and medicinal properties for centuries. Some studies suggest that saffron may have aphrodisiac effects, enhancing sexual desire and satisfaction.

20. Nutmeg: Nutmeg is a spice that has been used in traditional medicine for its medicinal properties. It contains compounds that may have aphrodisiac effects and improve sexual function.

21. Basil: Basil is an aromatic herb rich in antioxidants and nutrients like vitamin K and manganese. It is believed to have a stimulating effect on the senses and may enhance arousal and sexual desire when consumed.

22. Fennel: Fennel is a plant with a licorice-like flavor and is known for its potential to improve digestion and freshen breath. It contains compounds like anethole, which may have estrogenic effects and contribute to increased libido, particularly in women.

23. Vanilla: Vanilla is a popular flavoring agent derived from the orchid plant. Its sweet and comforting aroma is believed to have a calming effect on the nervous system,

Copyrighted material

potentially reducing stress and anxiety and promoting a relaxed state conducive to intimacy.

24. Cardamom: Cardamom is a spice commonly used in culinary dishes and traditional medicine. It is rich in antioxidants and essential oils that may promote blood flow and circulation, potentially enhancing sexual function and arousal.

25. Saffron: Saffron, derived from the stigma of the Crocus sativus flower, is one of the most expensive spices in the world. It has a long history of use as a culinary ingredient and medicinal herb. Saffron contains compounds like crocin and safranal, which may have mood-enhancing effects and contribute to increased libido and sexual pleasure.

26. Garlic: Garlic is a pungent herb known for its potential cardiovascular benefits and immune-boosting properties. It contains allicin, a compound that may improve blood circulation and overall cardiovascular health, potentially supporting erectile function and sexual performance.

27. Asparagus: Asparagus is a nutrient-rich vegetable packed with vitamins, minerals, and antioxidants. It is a natural source of folate, a B vitamin that plays a role in the production of histamine, a neurotransmitter involved in sexual arousal. Asparagus may also support hormone regulation and sexual function.

Copyrighted material

28. Cloves: Cloves are aromatic flower buds commonly used as a spice in cooking and traditional medicine. They contain eugenol, a compound with antioxidant and anti-inflammatory properties that may improve blood flow and circulation, potentially enhancing sexual function and arousal.

29. Pears: Pears are sweet and juicy fruits rich in fiber, vitamins, and antioxidants. They contain boron, a mineral that may support hormone regulation and sexual function. Pears also have a sensual texture and flavor that can be incorporated into romantic meals.

30. Pine Nuts: Pine nuts are nutrient-dense seeds rich in zinc, magnesium, and essential fatty acids. These nutrients are important for hormone production and cardiovascular health, supporting overall sexual function and vitality.

Incorporating a variety of these foods into your diet, along with maintaining a healthy lifestyle, may help support sexual health and enhance libido and sexual function. Remember that individual responses to these foods may vary, and it's essential to prioritize overall well-being for optimal sexual vitality.

Recipes and tips for incorporating aphrodisiacs into daily diet

1. Oyster Rockefeller Salad:

Copyrighted material

Ingredients:

- Fresh oysters
- Spinach leaves
- Butter
- Minced garlic
- Bread crumbs
- Parmesan cheese
- Lemon wedges

Instructions:

1. Preheat your oven to 450°F (232°C).
2. In a skillet, melt butter over medium heat and sauté minced garlic until fragrant.
3. Add bread crumbs and cook until golden brown.
4. Place spinach leaves on a baking sheet and arrange fresh oysters on top.
5. Spoon the garlic-breadcrumb mixture over the oysters and sprinkle with grated Parmesan cheese.
6. Bake in the preheated oven for about 8-10 minutes or until the oysters are cooked through.
7. Serve with lemon wedges for added flavor.

Copyrighted material

Tips: Oysters are rich in zinc, which is essential for testosterone production. Spinach is also high in magnesium, another mineral that supports healthy testosterone levels.

2. Chocolate-Covered Strawberries:

Ingredients:

- Fresh strawberries

- Dark chocolate chips

- Coconut oil

Instructions:

1. Wash and dry fresh strawberries, leaving the stems intact.

2. In a microwave-safe bowl, melt dark chocolate chips with a tablespoon of coconut oil in 30-second intervals, stirring until smooth.

3. Dip each strawberry into the melted chocolate, coating it halfway.

4. Place the chocolate-covered strawberries on a parchment-lined baking sheet and refrigerate until the chocolate sets.

5. Serve as a romantic dessert or snack.

Copyrighted material

Tips: Dark chocolate contains phenylethylamine, a compound that stimulates the release of endorphins and promotes feelings of pleasure and arousal. Strawberries are also rich in antioxidants, which support cardiovascular health and improve blood flow.

3. Ginseng Ginger Tea:

Ingredients:

- Fresh ginger root, sliced

- Ginseng tea bags or ginseng powder

- Honey (optional)

Instructions:

1. Bring a pot of water to a boil and add sliced ginger root.

2. Simmer for 10-15 minutes to infuse the water with ginger flavor.

3. Remove the pot from heat and add ginseng tea bags or ginseng powder.

4. Steep for an additional 5-10 minutes, depending on desired strength.

5. Strain the tea and sweeten with honey if desired.

6. Serve hot and enjoy as a soothing and invigorating beverage.

Copyrighted material

Tips: Ginger is known for its warming properties and may help increase blood circulation, while ginseng is believed to improve energy levels and enhance libido.

4. Saffron-infused Rice Pilaf:

Ingredients:

- Basmati rice

- Saffron threads

- Chicken or vegetable broth

- Chopped onions

- Chopped garlic

- Olive oil

- Chopped parsley or cilantro for garnish

Instructions:

1. Rinse basmati rice under cold water until the water runs clear. Drain and set aside.

2. In a large saucepan, heat olive oil over medium heat and sauté chopped onions and garlic until softened.

3. Add the rinsed rice to the saucepan and cook for a few minutes until lightly toasted.

Copyrighted material

4. In a separate bowl, steep saffron threads in warm chicken or vegetable broth until the liquid turns golden yellow.

5. Pour the saffron-infused broth over the rice and stir to combine.

6. Cover the saucepan and simmer over low heat for 15-20 minutes or until the rice is cooked through.

7. Fluff the rice with a fork and garnish with chopped parsley or cilantro before serving.

Tips: Saffron contains compounds like crocin and safranal, which may have mood-enhancing effects and contribute to increased libido and sexual pleasure.

5. Honey-Garlic Grilled Salmon:

Ingredients:

- Salmon fillets
- Minced garlic
- Honey
- Soy sauce
- Olive oil
- Lemon juice
- Salt and pepper to taste

Copyrighted material

Instructions:

1. In a bowl, whisk together minced garlic, honey, soy sauce, olive oil, lemon juice, salt, and pepper to create a marinade.

2. Place salmon fillets in a shallow dish and pour the marinade over them, ensuring they are well coated.

3. Cover and refrigerate for at least 30 minutes to allow the flavors to meld.

4. Preheat your grill to medium-high heat and lightly oil the grates.

5. Remove the salmon fillets from the marinade and grill for 4-5 minutes per side or until cooked through and lightly charred.

6. Serve the grilled salmon with a side of saffron-infused rice pilaf for a delicious and romantic meal.

Tips: Salmon is rich in omega-3 fatty acids, which support cardiovascular health and improve blood flow. Honey is a natural sweetener and may increase energy levels, while garlic contains allicin, a compound that may improve blood circulation and overall sexual function.

6. Spicy Avocado Chocolate Mousse:

Ingredients:

Copyrighted material

- Ripe avocados

- Dark chocolate chips

- Honey or maple syrup

- Cayenne pepper

- Cinnamon

- Vanilla extract

Instructions:

1. Melt dark chocolate chips in a microwave-safe bowl in 30-second intervals until smooth.

2. In a blender or food processor, combine ripe avocados, melted chocolate, honey or maple syrup, a pinch of cayenne pepper, a dash of cinnamon, and a splash of vanilla extract.

3. Blend until smooth and creamy, adjusting sweetness and spice to taste.

4. Divide the avocado chocolate mousse into serving dishes and refrigerate for at least 30 minutes to chill.

5. Serve chilled, garnished with a sprinkle of cinnamon or a dollop of whipped cream, if desired.

Copyrighted material

Tips: Avocados are rich in healthy fats and vitamins, while dark chocolate contains compounds that promote feelings of pleasure and arousal. The addition of spices like cayenne pepper and cinnamon adds a unique and stimulating flavor profile to this decadent dessert.

7. Maca Banana Smoothie:

Ingredients:

- Ripe bananas

- Almond milk or coconut milk

- Maca powder

- Honey or agave syrup

- Ice cubes (optional)

Instructions:

1. In a blender, combine ripe bananas, almond milk or coconut milk, a spoonful of maca powder, and a drizzle of honey or agave syrup.

2. Add ice cubes if desired and blend until smooth and creamy.

3. Pour the maca banana smoothie into glasses and serve immediately.

Tips: Maca root is known for its potential to increase libido and enhance sexual function. Combined with the

Copyrighted material

natural sweetness of bananas and the creaminess of almond milk or coconut milk, this smoothie makes a delicious and energizing treat.

8. Ginger-Lime Grilled Chicken:

Ingredients:

- Chicken breasts or thighs

- Fresh ginger, grated

- Lime zest and juice

- Garlic, minced

- Soy sauce or tamari

- Olive oil

- Salt and pepper

Instructions:

1. In a bowl, whisk together grated fresh ginger, lime zest, lime juice, minced garlic, soy sauce or tamari, olive oil, salt, and pepper to create a marinade.

2. Place chicken breasts or thighs in a shallow dish and pour the marinade over them, ensuring they are well coated.

3. Cover and refrigerate for at least 30 minutes to allow the flavors to meld.

Copyrighted material

4. Preheat your grill to medium-high heat and lightly oil the grates.

5. Remove the chicken from the marinade and grill for 6-8 minutes per side or until cooked through and lightly charred.

6. Serve the ginger-lime grilled chicken with a side of quinoa or wild rice for a satisfying and flavorful meal.

Tips: Ginger is known for its warming properties and may help increase blood circulation, while lime adds a refreshing citrus flavor to the grilled chicken. Pairing this dish with quinoa or wild rice provides a nutritious and hearty accompaniment.

9. Cinnamon-Spiced Roasted Carrots:

Ingredients:

- Carrots, peeled and halved lengthwise
- Olive oil
- Ground cinnamon
- Maple syrup
- Salt and pepper

Instructions:

1. Preheat your oven to 400°F (200°C).

Copyrighted material

2. Place halved carrots on a baking sheet and drizzle with olive oil.

3. Sprinkle ground cinnamon over the carrots, then drizzle with maple syrup.

4. Season with salt and pepper to taste.

5. Roast in the preheated oven for 20-25 minutes or until carrots are tender and caramelized.

6. Serve as a flavorful and aromatic side dish.

Tips: Cinnamon is believed to have stimulating effects and may enhance arousal. Paired with sweet maple syrup and the natural sweetness of roasted carrots, this dish makes a delicious and nutritious addition to any meal.

10. Vanilla Bean Panna Cotta:

Ingredients:

- Heavy cream

- Whole milk

- Granulated sugar

- Vanilla bean

- Gelatin powder

- Water

Instructions:

Copyrighted material

1. In a saucepan, combine heavy cream, whole milk, and granulated sugar.

2. Split a vanilla bean lengthwise and scrape the seeds into the cream mixture.

3. Heat the mixture over medium heat until it begins to simmer, then remove from heat.

4. In a small bowl, sprinkle gelatin powder over cold water and let it bloom for 5 minutes.

5. Whisk the bloomed gelatin into the warm cream mixture until fully dissolved.

6. Strain the mixture through a fine-mesh sieve to remove any vanilla bean seeds.

7. Pour the mixture into serving glasses or molds and refrigerate for at least 4 hours or until set.

8. Serve the vanilla bean panna cotta chilled, garnished with fresh berries or a drizzle of honey.

Tips: Vanilla is known for its sweet and comforting aroma, which can evoke feelings of relaxation and pleasure. This creamy and indulgent dessert is perfect for a romantic dinner or special occasion.

11. Sautéed Spinach with Garlic and Chili Flakes:

Ingredients:

- Fresh spinach leaves

Copyrighted material

- Olive oil

- Garlic cloves, thinly sliced

- Red chili flakes

- Lemon zest

- Salt and pepper

Instructions:

1. Heat olive oil in a skillet over medium heat.

2. Add thinly sliced garlic cloves and red chili flakes to the skillet and sauté until fragrant.

3. Add fresh spinach leaves to the skillet and toss until wilted.

4. Season with lemon zest, salt, and pepper to taste.

5. Remove from heat and serve immediately as a vibrant and flavorful side dish.

Tips: Spinach is high in magnesium, a mineral that supports healthy testosterone levels. Garlic and chili flakes add bold flavors to this quick and easy dish, making it a perfect accompaniment to any main course.

12. Romantic Raspberry Bellini:

Ingredients:

- Fresh raspberries

Copyrighted material

- Prosecco or champagne

- Raspberry liqueur (optional)

- Mint leaves for garnish

Instructions:

1. In a blender, purée fresh raspberries until smooth.

2. Strain the raspberry purée through a fine-mesh sieve to remove the seeds.

3. Pour the strained raspberry purée into champagne flutes, filling each glass halfway.

4. Top off each glass with chilled prosecco or champagne.

5. Add a splash of raspberry liqueur if desired for extra sweetness and flavor.

6. Garnish with fresh mint leaves and serve immediately.

Tips: Raspberries are rich in antioxidants and add a burst of color and flavor to this elegant cocktail. Paired with bubbly prosecco or champagne, this raspberry bellini is perfect for toasting to a romantic evening together.

13. Honey-Glazed Salmon with Asparagus:

Ingredients:

Copyrighted material

- Salmon fillets

- Honey

- Soy sauce

- Garlic cloves, minced

- Fresh lemon juice

- Olive oil

- Asparagus spears

- Salt and pepper

Instructions:

1. Preheat your oven to 400°F (200°C).

2. In a small bowl, whisk together honey, soy sauce, minced garlic, and fresh lemon juice to create the glaze.

3. Place salmon fillets on a baking sheet lined with parchment paper.

4. Brush the honey glaze over the salmon fillets, ensuring they are well coated.

5. Arrange asparagus spears around the salmon on the baking sheet.

6. Drizzle asparagus spears with olive oil and season with salt and pepper.

Copyrighted material

7. Bake in the preheated oven for 12-15 minutes or until salmon is cooked through and asparagus is tender.

8. Serve the honey-glazed salmon and asparagus hot, garnished with fresh lemon slices.

Tips: Honey is a natural sweetener that adds a touch of sweetness to the savory salmon fillets. Asparagus is rich in folate, which supports hormone production and may enhance sexual function.

14. Saffron Risotto with Shrimp:

Ingredients:

- Arborio rice

- Saffron threads

- Chicken or vegetable broth

- Shallots, finely chopped

- White wine

- Unsalted butter

- Parmesan cheese, grated

- Large shrimp, peeled and deveined

- Olive oil

- Salt and pepper

Copyrighted material

Instructions:

1. In a small bowl, steep saffron threads in warm chicken or vegetable broth until the liquid turns golden yellow.

2. In a saucepan, heat olive oil over medium heat and sauté finely chopped shallots until translucent.

3. Add Arborio rice to the saucepan and toast for a few minutes until lightly golden.

4. Pour white wine into the saucepan and stir until absorbed by the rice.

5. Gradually add the saffron-infused broth to the rice, stirring constantly until the rice is creamy and al dente.

6. Stir in unsalted butter and grated Parmesan cheese until melted and combined.

7. In a separate skillet, heat olive oil over medium-high heat and sauté peeled and deveined shrimp until pink and cooked through.

8. Serve the saffron risotto topped with sautéed shrimp, garnished with additional Parmesan cheese and freshly ground black pepper.

Tips: Saffron adds a luxurious and aromatic flavor to the creamy risotto, while shrimp provides a source of lean

Copyrighted material

protein. This dish is perfect for a romantic dinner at home.

15. Chocolate-Dipped Banana Bites:

Ingredients:

- Bananas, peeled and sliced into rounds

- Dark chocolate chips

- Coconut oil

- Assorted toppings (e.g., chopped nuts, shredded coconut, dried fruit)

Instructions:

1. Line a baking sheet with parchment paper.

2. In a microwave-safe bowl, melt dark chocolate chips with coconut oil in 30-second intervals until smooth.

3. Dip each banana slice halfway into the melted chocolate, then place it on the prepared baking sheet.

4. Sprinkle assorted toppings over the chocolate-dipped banana bites.

5. Place the baking sheet in the refrigerator for 15-20 minutes or until the chocolate sets.

Copyrighted material

6. Serve the chocolate-dipped banana bites chilled as a sweet and indulgent dessert.

Tips: Dark chocolate contains compounds that promote feelings of pleasure and arousal, while bananas provide natural sweetness and a creamy texture. Customize these chocolate-dipped banana bites with your favorite toppings for a delightful treat.

16. Spiced Hot Chocolate with Whipped Cream:

Ingredients:

- Milk (dairy or non-dairy)

- Dark chocolate, chopped

- Ground cinnamon

- Ground nutmeg

- Ground cayenne pepper

- Vanilla extract

- Whipped cream

- Cocoa powder for garnish

Instructions:

1. In a saucepan, heat milk over medium heat until warm but not boiling.

Copyrighted material

2. Add chopped dark chocolate to the warm milk and whisk until melted and smooth.

3. Stir in ground cinnamon, ground nutmeg, ground cayenne pepper, and vanilla extract to taste.

4. Pour the spiced hot chocolate into mugs and top each serving with a dollop of whipped cream.

5. Garnish with a sprinkle of cocoa powder before serving.

Tips: The combination of spices like cinnamon, nutmeg, and cayenne pepper adds a warming and aromatic flavor to the rich hot chocolate. Top with fluffy whipped cream for a decadent finishing touch.

17. Balsamic Glazed Fig and Prosciutto Crostini:

Ingredients:

- Baguette, sliced

- Fresh figs, sliced

- Prosciutto slices

- Balsamic glaze

- Goat cheese

- Fresh thyme leaves

- Olive oil

Copyrighted material

- Salt and pepper

Instructions:

1. Preheat your oven to 400°F (200°C).

2. Brush baguette slices with olive oil and arrange them on a baking sheet.

3. Toast baguette slices in the preheated oven for 5-7 minutes or until golden brown and crispy.

4. Spread goat cheese on each toasted baguette slice.

5. Top with sliced fresh figs and prosciutto slices.

6. Drizzle balsamic glaze over the fig and prosciutto crostini.

7. Garnish with fresh thyme leaves and season with salt and pepper to taste.

8. Serve as an elegant appetizer or hors d'oeuvre.

Tips: The combination of sweet figs, savory prosciutto, tangy goat cheese, and balsamic glaze creates a perfect balance of flavors in this sophisticated crostini.

18. Rosemary and Garlic Roasted Lamb Chops:

Ingredients:

- Lamb chops

Copyrighted material

- Fresh rosemary sprigs

- Garlic cloves, minced

- Olive oil

- Lemon zest

- Salt and pepper

Instructions:

1. Preheat your oven to 400°F (200°C).

2. Rub lamb chops with minced garlic, olive oil, lemon zest, and chopped fresh rosemary.

3. Season lamb chops with salt and pepper to taste.

4. Place lamb chops on a baking sheet lined with parchment paper.

5. Roast in the preheated oven for 12-15 minutes or until cooked to your desired doneness.

6. Remove from the oven and let the lamb chops rest for a few minutes before serving.

7. Serve the rosemary and garlic roasted lamb chops hot, garnished with additional fresh rosemary sprigs.

Tips: Rosemary and garlic add aromatic flavor to tender and juicy lamb chops, creating a delicious and elegant main course for a romantic dinner.

Copyrighted material

19. Mango Tango Smoothie Bowl:

Ingredients:

- Ripe mango, diced

- Frozen banana, sliced

- Greek yogurt or coconut yogurt

- Almond milk or coconut milk

- Honey or agave syrup

- Fresh lime juice

- Toppings: sliced kiwi, strawberries, granola, shredded coconut

Instructions:

1. In a blender, combine diced ripe mango, frozen banana slices, Greek yogurt or coconut yogurt, almond milk or coconut milk, honey or agave syrup, and fresh lime juice.

2. Blend until smooth and creamy, adding more almond milk or coconut milk if needed to reach your desired consistency.

3. Pour the mango smoothie into a bowl.

4. Arrange sliced kiwi, strawberries, granola, and shredded coconut on top of the mango smoothie.

Copyrighted material

5. Serve the mango tango smoothie bowl immediately for a refreshing and nutritious breakfast or snack.

Tips: The combination of sweet mango, tangy lime juice, and creamy yogurt creates a tropical and vibrant smoothie bowl that's as delicious as it is nutritious.

20. Grilled Pineapple with Honey-Lime Glaze:

Ingredients:

- Fresh pineapple, peeled and sliced into rings

- Honey

- Fresh lime juice

- Ground cinnamon

- Mint leaves for garnish

Instructions:

1. Preheat your grill to medium-high heat.

2. In a small bowl, whisk together honey, fresh lime juice, and ground cinnamon to create the glaze.

3. Brush both sides of pineapple rings with the honey-lime glaze.

4. Grill pineapple rings for 2-3 minutes per side or until grill marks appear and pineapple is caramelized.

Copyrighted material

5. Remove grilled pineapple from the grill and let it cool slightly.

6. Serve the grilled pineapple with a garnish of fresh mint leaves.

Tips: Grilling pineapple caramelizes its natural sugars and enhances its sweetness. The honey-lime glaze adds a tangy and aromatic flavor to this simple yet impressive dessert or side dish.

21. Lemon Garlic Shrimp Scampi:

Ingredients:

- Shrimp, peeled and deveined
- Linguine pasta
- Butter
- Olive oil
- Garlic cloves, minced
- Lemon juice and zest
- White wine
- Red pepper flakes
- Fresh parsley, chopped
- Salt and pepper

Instructions:

Copyrighted material

1. Cook linguine pasta according to package instructions until al dente. Drain and set aside.

2. In a large skillet, melt butter with olive oil over medium heat.

3. Add minced garlic and cook until fragrant.

4. Add shrimp to the skillet and cook until pink and opaque.

5. Stir in lemon juice, lemon zest, white wine, and red pepper flakes.

6. Toss cooked linguine with the shrimp mixture in the skillet.

7. Season with salt and pepper to taste and sprinkle with chopped parsley before serving.

Tips: The combination of garlic, lemon, and white wine creates a flavorful sauce that coats the tender shrimp and pasta, making this dish a perfect balance of tangy and savory flavors.

22. Caprese Salad with Balsamic Glaze:

Ingredients:

- Fresh mozzarella cheese, sliced

- Fresh tomatoes, sliced

- Fresh basil leaves

Copyrighted material

- Balsamic glaze

- Extra virgin olive oil

- Salt and pepper

Instructions:

1. Arrange sliced fresh mozzarella cheese, tomatoes, and basil leaves on a serving platter.

2. Drizzle with balsamic glaze and extra virgin olive oil.

3. Season with salt and pepper to taste before serving.

Tips: This classic Italian salad showcases the vibrant colors and flavors of fresh tomatoes, creamy mozzarella cheese, and fragrant basil, with a drizzle of tangy balsamic glaze adding a touch of sweetness.

23. Mediterranean Quinoa Salad:

Ingredients:

- Quinoa, cooked and cooled

- Cucumber, diced

- Cherry tomatoes, halved

- Kalamata olives, pitted and sliced

- Red onion, thinly sliced

Copyrighted material

- Feta cheese, crumbled

- Fresh parsley, chopped

- Lemon juice

- Extra virgin olive oil

- Salt and pepper

Instructions:

1. In a large bowl, combine cooked and cooled quinoa with diced cucumber, halved cherry tomatoes, sliced Kalamata olives, thinly sliced red onion, crumbled feta cheese, and chopped fresh parsley.

2. Drizzle with lemon juice and extra virgin olive oil.

3. Season with salt and pepper to taste and toss until well combined before serving.

Tips: This refreshing and nutritious salad is packed with Mediterranean flavors, including tangy feta cheese, briny olives, and fresh herbs, making it a perfect side dish or light meal option.

24. Stuffed Bell Peppers with Quinoa and Black Beans:

Ingredients:

- Bell peppers, halved and seeds removed

- Cooked quinoa

Copyrighted material

- Cooked black beans

- Corn kernels

- Diced tomatoes

- Red onion, diced

- Garlic, minced

- Chili powder

- Cumin

- Paprika

- Shredded cheese (optional)

- Fresh cilantro, chopped

- Lime wedges

Instructions:

1. Preheat your oven to 375°F (190°C).

2. In a large bowl, mix cooked quinoa, cooked black beans, corn kernels, diced tomatoes, diced red onion, minced garlic, chili powder, cumin, and paprika.

3. Stuff the halved bell peppers with the quinoa and black bean mixture.

4. Place stuffed bell peppers in a baking dish and sprinkle with shredded cheese if desired.

Copyrighted material

5. Cover the baking dish with aluminum foil and bake in the preheated oven for 25-30 minutes or until the bell peppers are tender.

6. Remove from the oven and garnish with chopped fresh cilantro and lime wedges before serving.

Tips: These colorful stuffed bell peppers are packed with protein-rich quinoa, fiber-packed black beans, and flavorful spices, making them a satisfying and wholesome meal option.

25. Mango Coconut Chia Pudding:

Ingredients:

- Chia seeds

- Coconut milk

- Mango, diced

- Coconut flakes

- Honey or agave syrup (optional)

Instructions:

1. In a bowl, mix chia seeds with coconut milk and diced mango.

2. Sweeten with honey or agave syrup if desired.

Copyrighted material

3. Cover and refrigerate for at least 4 hours or overnight until the chia seeds absorb the liquid and thicken into a pudding-like consistency.

4. Serve chilled, garnished with coconut flakes.

Tips: This tropical-inspired chia pudding combines the natural sweetness of ripe mangoes with creamy coconut milk and crunchy coconut flakes, creating a delicious and nutritious dessert or breakfast option.

26. Pesto Chicken Stuffed Sweet Potatoes:

Ingredients:

- Sweet potatoes

- Cooked chicken breast, shredded

- Pesto sauce

- Cherry tomatoes, halved

- Fresh basil leaves

- Parmesan cheese, grated

- Salt and pepper

Instructions:

1. Preheat your oven to 400°F (200°C).

2. Pierce sweet potatoes with a fork and bake in the preheated oven for 45-50 minutes or until tender.

Copyrighted material

3. Slice each sweet potato lengthwise and fluff the flesh with a fork.

4. Fill each sweet potato with shredded cooked chicken breast, pesto sauce, halved cherry tomatoes, fresh basil leaves, and grated Parmesan cheese.

5. Season with salt and pepper to taste before serving.

Tips: These hearty and flavorful stuffed sweet potatoes are filled with protein-packed chicken, aromatic pesto sauce, and fresh herbs, making them a satisfying and nutritious meal option.

27. Sautéed Garlic Butter Green Beans:

Ingredients:

- Green beans, trimmed

- Butter

- Olive oil

- Garlic cloves, minced

- Lemon zest

- Salt and pepper

Instructions:

Copyrighted material

1. In a large skillet, melt butter with olive oil over medium heat.

2. Add minced garlic to the skillet and cook until fragrant.

3. Add trimmed green beans to the skillet and sauté until crisp-tender.

4. Stir in lemon zest and season with salt and pepper to taste before serving.

Tips: This simple yet flavorful side dish features tender-crisp green beans sautéed with garlic-infused butter and bright lemon zest, making it a perfect accompaniment to any meal.

Copyrighted material

Chapter 4: Nutrition for Fertility

Importance of diet for fertility

The importance of diet for fertility cannot be overstated, as it plays a crucial role in both male and female reproductive health. A well-balanced diet rich in essential nutrients can significantly impact fertility by supporting hormonal balance, reproductive function, and overall reproductive health. Here are some key points highlighting the importance of diet for fertility:

1. Nutrient Intake: Adequate intake of essential nutrients such as vitamins, minerals, antioxidants, and omega-3 fatty acids is vital for reproductive health. These nutrients play various roles in hormone regulation, sperm and egg development, and overall reproductive function.

2. Hormonal Balance: Hormonal imbalances can adversely affect fertility in both men and women. A diet that supports hormonal balance can help regulate menstrual cycles, ovulation, sperm production, and sperm quality. Key nutrients involved in hormone regulation include vitamin D, vitamin E, zinc, selenium, and omega-3 fatty acids.

3. Body Weight: Maintaining a healthy body weight is essential for fertility. Both underweight and overweight individuals may experience fertility

Copyrighted material

issues due to hormonal imbalances. A balanced diet that supports a healthy weight can optimize fertility outcomes.

4. Blood Sugar Regulation: Stable blood sugar levels are important for fertility, as fluctuations in blood sugar levels can affect hormone levels and ovulation in women and sperm quality in men. Consuming complex carbohydrates, fiber, and protein-rich foods can help regulate blood sugar levels and support fertility.

5. Inflammation: Chronic inflammation in the body can impact fertility by affecting hormone levels and reproductive function. A diet rich in anti-inflammatory foods such as fruits, vegetables, whole grains, healthy fats, and lean proteins can help reduce inflammation and support fertility.

6. Antioxidants: Antioxidants play a crucial role in protecting reproductive cells from oxidative damage caused by free radicals. Consuming a diet rich in antioxidants from fruits, vegetables, nuts, seeds, and whole grains can help improve fertility outcomes by reducing oxidative stress.

7. Healthy Fats: Healthy fats, particularly omega-3 fatty acids found in fatty fish, flaxseeds, chia seeds, and walnuts, are important for reproductive health. Omega-3 fatty acids

Copyrighted material

contribute to hormone production, sperm development, and egg quality.

8. Hydration: Adequate hydration is essential for fertility as it supports overall health and helps maintain optimal cervical mucus production, which is important for sperm motility and transport.

9. Avoidance of Harmful Substances: Avoiding or minimizing the consumption of harmful substances such as alcohol, caffeine, tobacco, and recreational drugs is important for fertility. These substances can negatively impact hormone levels, sperm quality, and reproductive function.

10. Individualized Approach: It's important to note that individual nutritional needs may vary based on factors such as age, gender, underlying health conditions, and fertility status. Consulting with a healthcare provider or fertility specialist can help individuals develop personalized dietary recommendations to optimize fertility outcomes.

In summary, adopting a healthy and balanced diet that includes a variety of nutrient-rich foods, supports hormonal balance, regulates blood sugar levels, reduces inflammation, and provides adequate hydration is essential for optimizing fertility in both men and women.

Copyrighted material

Foods that promote reproductive health

Foods that promote reproductive health are rich in essential nutrients that support hormonal balance, reproductive function, and overall fertility. Incorporating a variety of nutrient-dense foods into your diet can provide the necessary vitamins, minerals, antioxidants, and healthy fats to optimize reproductive health. Here are some foods that are particularly beneficial for promoting reproductive health:

1. Leafy Green Vegetables: Leafy greens such as spinach, kale, Swiss chard, and collard greens are rich in folate, a B-vitamin that is essential for reproductive health. Folate supports sperm production in men and may improve fertility outcomes in women by promoting ovulation and reducing the risk of neural tube defects during pregnancy.

2. Berries: Berries like strawberries, blueberries, raspberries, and blackberries are packed with antioxidants such as vitamin C, anthocyanins, and flavonoids. These antioxidants help protect reproductive cells from oxidative damage caused by free radicals, thereby supporting fertility in both men and women.

3. Fatty Fish: Fatty fish such as salmon, mackerel, sardines, and trout are excellent sources of omega-3 fatty acids, particularly EPA and DHA.

Copyrighted material

Omega-3 fatty acids are essential for sperm development, sperm motility, and overall reproductive health. They also support hormonal balance and may improve fertility outcomes in women.

4. Nuts and Seeds: Nuts and seeds like almonds, walnuts, flaxseeds, and chia seeds are rich in healthy fats, protein, and antioxidants. They provide essential nutrients such as zinc, selenium, and vitamin E, which are important for sperm production, sperm quality, and reproductive function in both men and women.

5. Whole Grains: Whole grains such as oats, quinoa, brown rice, and barley are rich in complex carbohydrates, fiber, and B-vitamins. These nutrients support hormonal balance, regulate blood sugar levels, and promote overall reproductive health.

6. Legumes: Legumes such as lentils, chickpeas, black beans, and kidney beans are excellent sources of plant-based protein, fiber, and folate. They provide essential nutrients that support hormonal balance, ovulation, and sperm production.

7. Avocado: Avocado is a nutrient-dense fruit rich in healthy monounsaturated fats, vitamin E, and

Copyrighted material

potassium. It supports hormonal balance, provides antioxidants, and may improve fertility outcomes in both men and women.

8. Greek Yogurt: Greek yogurt is a rich source of protein, calcium, and probiotics. Protein supports sperm production and reproductive function, while calcium is important for ovarian function and hormone regulation. Probiotics promote gut health, which is linked to improved fertility outcomes.

9. Eggs: Eggs are a nutrient-rich source of protein, vitamin D, and choline. Vitamin D is important for hormonal balance and may improve fertility outcomes in both men and women. Choline supports fetal brain development during pregnancy.

10. Dark Chocolate: Dark chocolate contains flavonoids and antioxidants that support cardiovascular health and improve blood flow. It may also promote feelings of pleasure and arousal, thereby enhancing sexual function and fertility.

Incorporating these nutrient-rich foods into your diet as part of a balanced and varied eating plan can help support reproductive health and optimize fertility outcomes. Additionally, staying hydrated, maintaining a

Copyrighted material

healthy weight, and avoiding excessive alcohol intake, smoking, and processed foods can further contribute to reproductive wellness.

Advice for couples trying to conceive

For couples trying to conceive, there are several pieces of advice and recommendations that can help optimize fertility and improve the chances of successful conception. Here are some key pieces of advice for couples on their fertility journey:

1. Maintain a Healthy Lifestyle: Both partners should strive to maintain a healthy lifestyle by eating a balanced diet, exercising regularly, getting enough sleep, and managing stress. A healthy lifestyle can positively impact fertility by promoting hormonal balance, maintaining a healthy weight, and supporting overall reproductive health.

2. Know Your Fertile Window: Understanding the menstrual cycle and identifying the fertile window—the days leading up to ovulation and the day of ovulation itself—can increase the likelihood of conception. Tracking menstrual cycles, monitoring basal body temperature, and using ovulation predictor kits can help determine the most fertile days of the month.

Copyrighted material

3. Optimize Timing of Intercourse: Couples should aim to have regular, unprotected intercourse during the fertile window to maximize the chances of conception. Having sex every 1-2 days during the fertile window can ensure that sperm are present in the reproductive tract when ovulation occurs.

4. Address Underlying Health Conditions: It's important for both partners to address any underlying health conditions that may affect fertility. Conditions such as polycystic ovary syndrome (PCOS), endometriosis, thyroid disorders, and low sperm count or quality in men can impact fertility and may require medical intervention.

5. Limit Exposure to Harmful Substances: Both partners should avoid exposure to harmful substances that can affect fertility, such as tobacco smoke, alcohol, recreational drugs, and certain medications. Smoking and excessive alcohol consumption can impair fertility in both men and women.

6. Maintain a Healthy Weight: Both overweight and underweight individuals may experience fertility issues. Maintaining a healthy weight through a balanced diet and regular exercise can optimize fertility outcomes for both partners.

Copyrighted material

7. Seek Medical Advice: Couples who have been trying to conceive for a year (or six months for women over 35) without success should consider seeking medical advice from a fertility specialist. A fertility evaluation can help identify any underlying issues and determine the most appropriate course of action.

8. Consider Preconception Health: Both partners should consider their preconception health and take steps to optimize it before trying to conceive. This may include taking prenatal vitamins with folic acid, managing chronic health conditions, and discussing any concerns with a healthcare provider.

9. Manage Stress: High levels of stress can negatively impact fertility by disrupting hormonal balance and menstrual cycles. Couples should practice stress-reducing techniques such as mindfulness, meditation, yoga, or counseling to manage stress levels during the fertility journey.

10. Stay Positive and Support Each Other: Trying to conceive can be emotionally challenging, and it's important for couples to stay positive and supportive of each other throughout the process. Seeking support from family, friends, or support groups can also be helpful in coping with the emotional aspects of fertility struggles.

Copyrighted material

By following these pieces of advice and recommendations, couples can optimize their fertility and improve their chances of successfully conceiving a healthy pregnancy. It's important to remember that fertility is a complex process influenced by various factors, and seeking guidance from healthcare professionals can provide valuable support and assistance along the way.

Copyrighted material

Chapter 5: Diet and Sexual Dysfunctions

Negative effects of poor diet on sexual dysfunctions. Poor diet can have significant negative effects on sexual dysfunctions in both men and women. A diet lacking in essential nutrients, high in unhealthy fats and sugars, and low in antioxidants and vitamins can contribute to various sexual dysfunctions. Here are some negative effects of poor diet on sexual dysfunctions:

1. Hormonal Imbalance: A diet high in processed foods, saturated fats, and sugars can disrupt hormonal balance, leading to imbalances in sex hormones such as testosterone, estrogen, and progesterone. Hormonal imbalances can contribute to sexual dysfunctions such as low libido, erectile dysfunction (ED) in men, and irregular menstrual cycles or decreased libido in women.

2. Obesity and Metabolic Syndrome: Poor diet characterized by excessive calorie intake, high levels of refined carbohydrates, and unhealthy fats can contribute to obesity and metabolic syndrome. Obesity is associated with sexual dysfunctions such as erectile dysfunction, reduced sexual desire, and difficulties with arousal and orgasm. Metabolic syndrome,

Copyrighted material

characterized by insulin resistance, high blood pressure, and abnormal cholesterol levels, can also negatively impact sexual function.

3. Cardiovascular Health: A diet high in saturated fats, trans fats, and cholesterol can contribute to cardiovascular diseases such as atherosclerosis, hypertension, and coronary artery disease. Poor cardiovascular health is closely linked to sexual dysfunctions such as erectile dysfunction, as adequate blood flow to the genital area is essential for achieving and maintaining an erection in men.

4. Diabetes and Insulin Resistance: Diets high in refined sugars and carbohydrates can contribute to insulin resistance and the development of type 2 diabetes. Diabetes is associated with sexual dysfunctions such as erectile dysfunction, decreased libido, and difficulties with arousal and orgasm. Poorly controlled diabetes can also lead to nerve damage (neuropathy) and vascular problems, further exacerbating sexual dysfunctions.

5. Inflammation and Oxidative Stress: Poor diet lacking in antioxidants and phytonutrients can contribute to chronic inflammation and oxidative stress in the body. Inflammation and oxidative stress are implicated in the pathogenesis of

Copyrighted material

various sexual dysfunctions, including erectile dysfunction and reduced sexual desire. Antioxidants play a crucial role in protecting reproductive cells from oxidative damage and maintaining overall sexual health.

6. Psychological Impact: Poor diet and unhealthy eating habits can have a negative impact on mental health, leading to conditions such as depression, anxiety, and stress. Psychological factors are closely linked to sexual dysfunctions, as they can affect sexual desire, arousal, and overall sexual satisfaction.

In summary, poor diet characterized by excessive intake of unhealthy fats, sugars, and processed foods, along with inadequate intake of essential nutrients, can have detrimental effects on sexual dysfunctions. Adopting a balanced diet rich in whole foods, fruits, vegetables, lean proteins, and healthy fats can help improve overall health and support sexual function and well-being. Additionally, addressing underlying health conditions and maintaining a healthy lifestyle are essential for preventing and managing sexual dysfunctions associated with poor diet and nutrition.

Foods that may worsen sexual dysfunctions

Certain foods may exacerbate sexual dysfunctions by contributing to hormonal imbalances, cardiovascular issues, inflammation, and other underlying health

Copyrighted material

conditions. Here are some foods that may worsen sexual dysfunctions:

1. Processed Foods: Processed foods high in refined sugars, unhealthy fats, and artificial additives can contribute to obesity, insulin resistance, and inflammation, all of which are risk factors for sexual dysfunctions such as erectile dysfunction (ED) and low libido.

2. High-Sodium Foods: Foods high in sodium, such as processed meats, canned soups, and fast food, can contribute to hypertension (high blood pressure) and cardiovascular problems, which can negatively impact sexual function.

3. Sugary Beverages: Sugary beverages like soda, energy drinks, and sweetened fruit juices can contribute to insulin resistance, weight gain, and metabolic syndrome, all of which are associated with sexual dysfunctions.

4. Fried Foods: Fried foods high in unhealthy fats, such as French fries, fried chicken, and doughnuts, can contribute to obesity, cardiovascular problems, and inflammation, which can affect sexual function.

5. Highly Processed Carbohydrates: Highly processed carbohydrates like white bread, pastries, and sugary cereals can cause rapid spikes

Copyrighted material

in blood sugar levels, leading to insulin resistance and metabolic issues that may worsen sexual dysfunctions.

6. Alcohol: Excessive alcohol consumption can impair sexual function by affecting hormonal balance, reducing testosterone levels, and interfering with sexual arousal and performance. Chronic alcohol abuse can also contribute to liver damage and neuropathy, which may further exacerbate sexual dysfunctions.

7. Caffeine: While moderate caffeine intake is generally considered safe, excessive consumption of caffeinated beverages like coffee, energy drinks, and certain teas can lead to anxiety, insomnia, and increased heart rate, which may negatively impact sexual function.

8. Highly Processed Meats: Highly processed meats like hot dogs, sausages, and deli meats often contain high levels of saturated fats, sodium, and additives, which can contribute to cardiovascular issues and inflammation associated with sexual dysfunctions.

9. Artificial Trans Fats: Foods containing artificial trans fats, such as margarine, fried foods, and commercially baked goods, can contribute to inflammation, oxidative stress, and

Copyrighted material

cardiovascular problems that may worsen sexual dysfunctions.

10. Excessive Red Meat: While lean cuts of red meat can be part of a healthy diet in moderation, excessive consumption of red meat, especially processed red meats like bacon and sausage, has been linked to cardiovascular issues and inflammation, which can impact sexual function.

It's important to note that individual responses to foods may vary, and what worsens sexual dysfunctions for one person may not affect another in the same way. However, reducing intake of the aforementioned foods and focusing on a balanced diet rich in whole foods, fruits, vegetables, lean proteins, and healthy fats may help improve overall health and support sexual function. Additionally, consulting with a healthcare provider or registered dietitian for personalized dietary recommendations is advisable for individuals experiencing sexual dysfunctions.

Dietary advice for addressing sexual dysfunctions

Addressing sexual dysfunctions through dietary changes involves adopting a balanced and nutritious diet that supports overall health and addresses underlying factors contributing to sexual issues. Here are some dietary recommendations for addressing sexual dysfunctions:

Copyrighted material

1. Eat a Balanced Diet: Consume a balanced diet that includes a variety of nutrient-dense foods from all food groups, including fruits, vegetables, whole grains, lean proteins, and healthy fats. Aim for a diet that provides essential vitamins, minerals, antioxidants, and phytonutrients to support overall health and sexual function.

2. Focus on Whole Foods: Choose whole, minimally processed foods over highly processed and refined foods. Whole foods are rich in nutrients and fiber and provide sustained energy levels, which can help support hormonal balance and overall well-being.

3. Increase Intake of Fruits and Vegetables: Incorporate a variety of fruits and vegetables into your diet, as they are rich in vitamins, minerals, antioxidants, and phytonutrients that support cardiovascular health, reduce inflammation, and improve blood flow—all of which are important for sexual function.

4. Include Lean Proteins: Choose lean sources of protein such as poultry, fish, beans, lentils, tofu, and Greek yogurt. Protein is essential for muscle health, hormone production, and overall energy levels, which can positively impact sexual function.

Copyrighted material

5. Healthy Fats: Include sources of healthy fats in your diet such as avocados, nuts, seeds, olive oil, and fatty fish like salmon and mackerel. Healthy fats support hormone production, brain health, and cardiovascular function, all of which are important for sexual health.

6. Whole Grains: Choose whole grains such as brown rice, quinoa, oats, and whole wheat bread over refined grains. Whole grains provide fiber, vitamins, and minerals that support heart health and blood sugar regulation, which are important for sexual function.

7. Stay Hydrated: Drink plenty of water throughout the day to stay hydrated. Proper hydration is important for overall health and supports blood circulation, which is essential for sexual arousal and function.

8. Limit Added Sugars and Processed Foods: Minimize consumption of foods and beverages high in added sugars, refined carbohydrates, unhealthy fats, and processed ingredients. These foods can contribute to inflammation, insulin resistance, and cardiovascular issues that may negatively impact sexual function.

9. Moderate Alcohol Consumption: If you consume alcohol, do so in moderation. Excessive alcohol

Copyrighted material

consumption can impair sexual function by affecting hormone levels, nervous system function, and cardiovascular health.

10. Consider Specific Nutrients: Some nutrients may have specific benefits for sexual health. For example, foods rich in zinc (such as oysters, beef, and pumpkin seeds) and magnesium (such as spinach, almonds, and dark chocolate) may support testosterone production and improve sexual function in men. Additionally, foods rich in antioxidants (such as berries, citrus fruits, and leafy greens) may help reduce oxidative stress and support overall sexual health.

It's important to remember that dietary changes alone may not completely resolve sexual dysfunctions, especially if there are underlying medical or psychological factors involved. Consulting with a healthcare provider or registered dietitian can provide personalized recommendations and support for addressing sexual dysfunctions through diet and lifestyle modifications. Additionally, addressing any underlying medical conditions and seeking appropriate medical treatment or counseling is important for managing sexual health issues effectively.

Copyrighted material

Chapter 6: Dietary Program to Enhance Sexual Health

Practical guide for a diet aimed at sexual health
Creating a practical guide for a diet aimed at improving sexual health involves incorporating nutrient-rich foods that support hormonal balance, cardiovascular health, and overall well-being. Here's a comprehensive guide with dietary advice for addressing sexual dysfunctions:

1. Focus on Whole Foods: Base your diet on whole, nutrient-dense foods such as fruits, vegetables, whole grains, lean proteins, and healthy fats. These foods provide essential vitamins, minerals, antioxidants, and phytonutrients that support sexual health.

2. Optimize Protein Intake: Include lean sources of protein such as poultry, fish, tofu, legumes, and nuts in your diet. Protein is essential for hormone production, muscle health, and overall energy levels.

3. Incorporate Healthy Fats: Include sources of healthy fats such as avocados, olive oil, nuts, seeds, and fatty fish like salmon and sardines. Healthy fats support hormonal balance, cardiovascular health, and reproductive function.

Copyrighted material

4. Prioritize Antioxidants: Consume foods rich in antioxidants such as berries, citrus fruits, leafy greens, and colorful vegetables. Antioxidants help protect reproductive cells from oxidative damage and support overall sexual health.

5. Include Omega-3 Fatty Acids: Incorporate omega-3 fatty acids from sources like fatty fish, flaxseeds, chia seeds, and walnuts. Omega-3s support cardiovascular health, reduce inflammation, and may improve sexual function.

6. Stay Hydrated: Drink plenty of water throughout the day to stay hydrated. Adequate hydration supports blood flow, lubrication, and overall sexual function.

7. Moderate Alcohol Consumption: Limit alcohol consumption as excessive intake can impair sexual function. If you choose to drink alcohol, do so in moderation and opt for red wine, which contains antioxidants like resveratrol.

8. Limit Added Sugars: Minimize consumption of foods and beverages high in added sugars, such as sugary snacks, desserts, and sweetened beverages. High sugar intake can contribute to inflammation and negatively impact sexual health.

Copyrighted material

9. Manage Caffeine Intake: Moderate caffeine consumption is generally fine, but excessive intake can contribute to anxiety and interfere with sexual arousal. Be mindful of your caffeine intake from sources like coffee, tea, and energy drinks.

10. Maintain a Healthy Weight: Aim to maintain a healthy weight through a balanced diet and regular physical activity. Excess weight can contribute to hormonal imbalances and cardiovascular issues that may impact sexual function.

11. Practice Portion Control: Pay attention to portion sizes to avoid overeating and maintain a healthy weight. Use smaller plates, eat slowly, and listen to your body's hunger and fullness cues.

12. Seek Professional Guidance: If you're experiencing sexual dysfunctions or have specific concerns about your diet and sexual health, consider seeking guidance from a healthcare provider or registered dietitian. They can provide personalized recommendations and support based on your individual needs.

By following these dietary guidelines and incorporating nutrient-rich foods into your daily meals, you can support hormonal balance, cardiovascular health, and overall

Copyrighted material

well-being, which are essential for optimal sexual health. Remember that consistency and balance are key, and making gradual changes to your diet can lead to long-term improvements in sexual function and overall health.

Meal preparation tips

Meal preparation is like setting the stage for a successful culinary journey throughout the week. Picture this: you carve out some time on a lazy Sunday afternoon, maybe with some background music playing, and you dive into prepping ingredients like a kitchen magician. It's not just about saving time; it's about setting yourself up for healthy eating habits and making life a bit easier when things get hectic.

So, how do we embark on this meal prep adventure? Well, it starts with a plan. Take a moment to think about what meals you'd like to enjoy during the week. Are there any favorite recipes you're itching to make or new ones you're excited to try? Jot them down and make a grocery list based on what you'll need.

Once you have your game plan, it's time to hit the kitchen. Get those veggies washed, chopped, and ready to go. Think colorful bell peppers, crisp lettuce, and vibrant tomatoes. Having them prepped and portioned means they're just a grab away when you're assembling a salad or stir-fry later in the week.

Copyrighted material

Next up, let's talk about batch cooking. This is where the magic happens. Whip up a big pot of quinoa or brown rice, grill some chicken breasts or tofu, and roast a medley of veggies all at once. Suddenly, you've got the building blocks for multiple meals. You can mix and match these ingredients throughout the week, whether it's tossing them into a Buddha bowl or layering them in a hearty grain salad.

Don't forget about breakfast! Overnight oats are a game-changer. Just mix oats, milk (or your favorite alternative), and toppings like fruits and nuts in a jar, pop it in the fridge, and wake up to a ready-to-eat breakfast. It's nutritious, delicious, and requires zero morning effort.

And let's not overlook snacks. Having healthy options like pre-portioned nuts, yogurt parfaits, or sliced veggies and hummus on hand can help curb those mid-afternoon cravings and keep you fueled throughout the day.

Oh, and labeling is your friend. Trust me, you don't want to play the guessing game when you open the fridge and find a mystery container. Labeling your meal prep containers with the date and contents keeps things organized and ensures nothing goes to waste.

Lastly, remember to keep it fun! Get creative with your recipes, experiment with different flavors and cuisines, and involve the whole family if you can. Meal prep doesn't have to be a chore; it can be a fun and rewarding

Copyrighted material

way to nourish your body and soul throughout the week. So, grab your apron and let's get prepping!

Strategies for maintaining a healthy diet long-term

Maintaining a healthy diet long-term requires a combination of mindful eating habits, realistic goals, and sustainable strategies. Here are some key strategies for sticking to a healthy diet over the long haul:

1. Focus on Whole Foods: Base your diet around whole, minimally processed foods such as fruits, vegetables, whole grains, lean proteins, and healthy fats. These foods are nutrient-dense and provide essential vitamins, minerals, and antioxidants to support overall health.

2. Practice Portion Control: Be mindful of portion sizes and avoid overeating, even when consuming healthy foods. Use smaller plates, pay attention to hunger and fullness cues, and aim for balanced meals that include a variety of food groups.

3. Moderation, Not Deprivation: Allow yourself to enjoy your favorite foods in moderation. Depriving yourself of foods you love can lead to feelings of deprivation and ultimately sabotage your efforts to maintain a healthy diet long-term. Instead, practice mindful indulgence and savor your treats occasionally.

Copyrighted material

4. Meal Planning and Preparation: Plan your meals ahead of time and prep ingredients in advance to make healthy eating more convenient. Batch cooking, portioning out meals, and having healthy snacks on hand can help you stay on track, even on busy days.

5. Set Realistic Goals: Set realistic, achievable goals for your diet and focus on making gradual, sustainable changes rather than aiming for perfection. Celebrate small victories along the way and acknowledge that progress takes time.

6. Listen to Your Body: Pay attention to how different foods make you feel and listen to your body's hunger and fullness cues. Eat when you're hungry and stop when you're satisfied, rather than eating out of boredom, stress, or emotions.

7. Stay Hydrated: Drink plenty of water throughout the day to stay hydrated and support overall health. Sometimes, thirst can be mistaken for hunger, so staying hydrated can help prevent unnecessary snacking.

8. Incorporate Variety: Keep your meals interesting and diverse by incorporating a variety of foods from different food groups, cuisines, and flavors. Experiment with new recipes, ingredients, and

Copyrighted material

cooking methods to keep your taste buds engaged.

9. Mindful Eating: Practice mindful eating by slowing down, savoring each bite, and paying attention to the sensory experience of eating. Avoid distractions such as screens or multitasking while eating, and focus on enjoying your food.

10. Be Kind to Yourself: Remember that nobody's perfect, and it's normal to have ups and downs on your journey to maintaining a healthy diet. Be kind to yourself, practice self-compassion, and don't be too hard on yourself if you have occasional slip-ups.

11. Seek Support: Surround yourself with a supportive environment that encourages healthy eating habits. This could include friends, family members, or online communities who share your goals and can provide encouragement and accountability.

12. Flexibility and Adaptability: Be flexible and adaptable with your diet, especially in social situations or when faced with unexpected challenges. Learning to navigate different situations while staying true to your long-term health goals is key to maintaining a healthy diet in the real world.

Copyrighted material

By incorporating these strategies into your lifestyle and mindset, you can cultivate healthy eating habits that last a lifetime. Remember that maintaining a healthy diet is not about perfection but rather about making consistent, sustainable choices that support your overall health and well-being.

Copyrighted material

Chapter 7: Supplements and Natural Remedies

Dietary supplements useful for improving sexual health.

Dietary supplements can play a role in supporting sexual health by providing essential nutrients and promoting overall well-being. While it's important to prioritize a balanced diet rich in whole foods, some supplements may offer additional benefits. Here are some dietary supplements that have been researched for their potential to improve sexual health:

1. L-arginine: L-arginine is an amino acid that plays a role in the production of nitric oxide, a compound that helps relax blood vessels and improve blood flow. It may help enhance erectile function in men by improving blood flow to the genital area.

2. Ginseng: Ginseng is an herb that has been used traditionally in Chinese medicine to improve vitality and sexual function. Some research suggests that ginseng may help improve erectile function and libido in men.

3. Maca: Maca root is a plant native to Peru that is often used as a natural aphrodisiac. Some studies have found that maca may help improve sexual

Copyrighted material

desire and erectile function in men, as well as reduce sexual dysfunction in women.

4. Fenugreek: Fenugreek is an herb commonly used in traditional medicine to enhance libido and sexual performance. It may help improve sexual function and testosterone levels in men.

5. Tribulus terrestris: Tribulus terrestris is a plant that has been used in traditional medicine to enhance libido and sexual function. Some research suggests that it may help improve erectile function and increase sexual desire in both men and women.

6. Zinc: Zinc is an essential mineral that plays a role in testosterone production and sperm health. Low levels of zinc have been associated with sexual dysfunction in men, so supplementation may be beneficial for those with deficiencies.

7. Vitamin D: Vitamin D is important for overall health and may also play a role in sexual function. Some studies have found an association between low vitamin D levels and sexual dysfunction in men, so supplementation may be helpful for those with deficiencies.

8. Omega-3 fatty acids: Omega-3 fatty acids, found in fish oil supplements, may help improve cardiovascular health and blood flow, which are

Copyrighted material

important for sexual function. Some research suggests that omega-3 fatty acids may also have a positive effect on libido and sexual satisfaction.

9. Ashwagandha: Ashwagandha is an herb commonly used in traditional Ayurvedic medicine to improve vitality and sexual function. Some studies have found that ashwagandha may help improve sexual desire, arousal, and satisfaction in both men and women.

10. L-citrulline: L-citrulline is an amino acid that is converted into L-arginine in the body, leading to increased production of nitric oxide. Some research suggests that L-citrulline supplementation may help improve erectile function in men with mild to moderate erectile dysfunction.

It's important to note that while some studies suggest potential benefits of these supplements for sexual health, more research is needed to fully understand their effectiveness and safety. Additionally, it's important to consult with a healthcare professional before starting any new supplement regimen, especially if you have underlying health conditions or are taking medications. A healthcare provider can help determine if a supplement is appropriate for you and provide guidance on proper dosage and potential interactions with other medications.

Copyrighted material

Natural remedies and herbs that can support sexual function

In addition to dietary supplements, certain natural remedies and herbs have been traditionally used to support sexual function. While scientific evidence on their effectiveness may vary, some individuals find these remedies helpful. Here are some natural remedies and herbs that may support sexual function:

Ginkgo Biloba: Ginkgo biloba is an herb that has been used in traditional medicine to improve blood circulation, which may benefit sexual function by enhancing blood flow to the genital area. Some studies suggest that ginkgo biloba may help improve erectile function and sexual satisfaction.

Horny Goat Weed (Epimedium): Horny goat weed is an herb that has been used in traditional Chinese medicine as an aphrodisiac. It contains compounds that may help improve sexual function by increasing blood flow and supporting hormonal balance. Some research suggests that horny goat weed may help improve erectile function and libido.

Tribulus Terrestris: Tribulus terrestris is a plant that has been used in traditional medicine to enhance libido and sexual performance. It contains compounds that may help increase testosterone levels and improve sexual function in both men and women.

Copyrighted material

Maca Root: Maca root is a plant native to Peru that has been used traditionally as an aphrodisiac and fertility enhancer. Some studies suggest that maca root may help improve sexual desire, erectile function, and sperm quality.

Ashwagandha: Ashwagandha is an herb commonly used in traditional Ayurvedic medicine to improve vitality and sexual function. It contains compounds that may help reduce stress and anxiety, which can have a positive effect on sexual function. Some research suggests that ashwagandha may help improve sexual desire, arousal, and satisfaction.

Damiana: Damiana is an herb native to Central and South America that has been used traditionally as an aphrodisiac and tonic for sexual health. It contains compounds that may help improve blood flow and stimulate sexual desire.

Yohimbe: Yohimbe is an herb derived from the bark of the yohimbe tree, native to West Africa. It has been used traditionally as an aphrodisiac and to treat erectile dysfunction. Yohimbe contains a compound called yohimbine, which may help improve sexual function by increasing blood flow to the genital area. However, it can have side effects and should be used with caution.

Saw Palmetto: Saw palmetto is a palm plant native to the southeastern United States. It has been used traditionally

Copyrighted material

to support prostate health and improve urinary function. Some research suggests that saw palmetto may also have benefits for sexual function by supporting hormonal balance.

Cacao: Cacao, the raw form of cocoa, contains compounds such as phenylethylamine (PEA) and anandamide, which are known as "feel-good" chemicals that can enhance mood and promote relaxation. Some people find that consuming cacao or dark chocolate can have a positive effect on sexual desire and pleasure.

Fenugreek: Fenugreek is an herb commonly used in traditional medicine to enhance libido and sexual performance. It contains compounds that may help improve sexual function and testosterone levels in men.

It's important to note that while some individuals may find these natural remedies and herbs helpful for supporting sexual function, scientific evidence on their effectiveness is limited and varies. Additionally, it's essential to consult with a healthcare professional before using any natural remedies or herbs, especially if you have underlying health conditions or are taking medications. A healthcare provider can help determine if these remedies are appropriate for you and provide guidance on proper usage and potential interactions with other medications.

Copyrighted material

Considerations regarding the safety and efficacy of supplements and remedies

When considering the safety and efficacy of supplements and remedies, it's crucial to approach them with a thoughtful and informed perspective. While some supplements and natural remedies may offer potential benefits, there are important considerations to keep in mind:

1. Scientific Evidence:

- Safety: The safety of a supplement or remedy should be supported by scientific evidence. Look for well-conducted clinical trials and studies that assess both short-term and long-term safety.

- Efficacy: The efficacy of a supplement or remedy refers to its ability to produce the desired effects. Look for scientific studies with robust methodologies that demonstrate effectiveness in addressing specific health concerns.

2. Regulatory Oversight:

- Supplement Regulation: Dietary supplements are not regulated as strictly as pharmaceutical drugs in many countries. Be cautious about claims made by supplement manufacturers, and choose products from reputable brands that adhere to quality and safety standards.

Copyrighted material

- Herbal Remedies: Herbal remedies may not undergo the same rigorous testing and regulatory scrutiny as pharmaceutical drugs. Consider consulting with a healthcare professional knowledgeable in herbal medicine for guidance.

3. Individual Variability:

- Body Response: Individuals can respond differently to supplements and remedies. Factors such as age, health status, medications, and genetic variations can influence how the body interacts with these substances.

- Underlying Conditions: If you have existing health conditions or are taking medications, it's crucial to consult with a healthcare provider before introducing supplements or remedies to your routine.

4. Potential Interactions:

- Medication Interactions: Some supplements and remedies may interact with medications, either enhancing or reducing their effectiveness. Always inform your healthcare provider about any supplements you are taking to avoid potential interactions.

Copyrighted material

- Combinations: Be cautious when combining multiple supplements, as the cumulative effects and interactions are not always well understood.

5. Dosage and Duration:

- Appropriate Dosage: Adhere to recommended dosages provided on the supplement or remedy packaging. Excessive doses may lead to adverse effects.

- Duration of Use: Some supplements and remedies are intended for short-term use, while others may be suitable for long-term use. Follow guidance on duration and consult with a healthcare professional for extended use.

6. Quality and Purity:

- Product Quality: Choose supplements from reputable manufacturers that adhere to quality standards. Look for products with third-party testing for purity and potency.

- Herbal Sourcing: For herbal remedies, consider the source of the herbs and how they are processed. Contamination and inconsistent concentrations can occur if quality control measures are not in place.

7. Health Professional Consultation:

Copyrighted material

- Consult Healthcare Professionals: Before incorporating supplements or remedies into your routine, consult with a qualified healthcare professional. They can provide personalized advice based on your health history and specific needs.

- Monitoring: Regularly monitor your health status and report any unexpected symptoms or changes to your healthcare provider.

8. Lifestyle Factors:

- Holistic Approach: Supplements and remedies should complement a healthy lifestyle, including a balanced diet, regular exercise, and stress management. They are not a substitute for overall well-being.

In summary, while supplements and remedies may have potential benefits, a cautious and informed approach is essential. Consult with healthcare professionals, prioritize evidence-based options, and consider individual factors for a well-rounded perspective on safety and efficacy.

Copyrighted material

Conclusion

Implementing a healthy diet for sexual health is not just about following a set of rules or restrictions—it's a journey of self-discovery and empowerment that encompasses various aspects of our lives. It's about making conscious choices that nourish our bodies, support our overall well-being, and enhance our sexual vitality.

One of the fundamental aspects of implementing a healthy diet for sexual health is focusing on balanced nutrition. This means incorporating a wide variety of nutrient-rich foods into our meals, including fruits, vegetables, whole grains, lean proteins, and healthy fats. These foods provide essential vitamins, minerals, and antioxidants that support optimal sexual function and overall health.

In addition to focusing on nutrient-rich foods, it's important to prioritize hydration. Drinking plenty of water throughout the day helps maintain proper blood flow, supports hormone balance, and ensures that our bodies are functioning optimally. Staying hydrated is crucial for sexual health, as dehydration can affect arousal and sexual performance.

Furthermore, minimizing the intake of processed foods, sugary snacks, and sugary drinks is key. These foods can contribute to inflammation, hormonal imbalances, and decreased sexual function. By choosing whole, minimally processed foods instead, we can provide our bodies with the nourishment they need to thrive.

Copyrighted material

Moderating alcohol consumption is another important aspect of implementing a healthy diet for sexual health. While alcohol can lower inhibitions and increase arousal in the short term, excessive alcohol consumption can impair sexual function and decrease libido over time. Finding a balance that works for you is essential for supporting sexual health.

Managing stress is also crucial for maintaining sexual health. Chronic stress can negatively impact hormone levels, increase tension in the body, and interfere with sexual function. Incorporating stress management techniques such as mindfulness, meditation, and deep breathing exercises into our daily routine can help us relax and reduce stress levels.

Regular physical activity is another important component of a healthy diet for sexual health. Exercise improves cardiovascular health, enhances blood flow, boosts mood and energy levels, and supports overall well-being—all of which contribute to sexual health. Finding activities that we enjoy and incorporating them into our routine can help us stay active and support our sexual vitality.

Finally, open and honest communication with our partner about our sexual health and needs is essential. Creating a supportive and understanding environment where we can discuss any concerns or desires openly is crucial for maintaining a healthy and fulfilling sex life. Working together to find solutions that support both partners' needs can strengthen the relationship and enhance sexual satisfaction.

Overall, implementing a healthy diet for sexual health is about more than just what we eat—it's about creating a lifestyle that supports our overall well-being and enhances our sexual

Copyrighted material

vitality. By focusing on balanced nutrition, hydration, stress management, physical activity, and open communication with our partner, we can create a supportive environment for sexual health and well-being.

In conclusion, "Sexual Power Diet" represents more than just a dietary guide—it embodies a holistic approach to sexual health and overall well-being. Throughout this journey, we've delved deep into the intricate interplay between nutrition and sexual vitality, uncovering the profound impact that dietary choices can have on our intimate lives.

By exploring the scientific underpinnings of how nutrients influence hormonal balance, libido, and sexual function, this book has provided readers with invaluable insights into the power of food to nourish not just our bodies, but also our relationships and sense of self. From understanding the role of antioxidants in protecting reproductive cells to discovering the aphrodisiacal properties of certain foods, "Sexual Power Diet" has equipped readers with the knowledge to make informed dietary decisions that support their sexual well-being.

Moreover, this book has sought to break down barriers and destigmatize discussions around sexual health, fostering an open and honest dialogue that empowers individuals to prioritize their intimate lives without shame or judgment. By addressing common misconceptions and societal taboos, "Sexual Power Diet" encourages readers to embrace their sexuality as an integral part of their overall health and happiness.

But "Sexual Power Diet" is more than just information—it's a call to action. It's an invitation for readers to embark on a

Copyrighted material

transformative journey of self-discovery and empowerment, where they can cultivate a deeper connection with their bodies, nurture intimate relationships, and embrace a more fulfilling and satisfying sexual life. Through practical advice, actionable strategies, and inspiring stories, this book serves as a roadmap for readers to reclaim their sexual power and live life to the fullest.

As we close this chapter, let us remember that the principles outlined in "Sexual Power Diet" are not just about what we eat, but how we choose to nourish ourselves—body, mind, and soul. May this book serve as a guiding light on your journey to sexual vitality and well-being, empowering you to embrace a lifestyle that honors and celebrates the incredible power of your sexuality.

Copyrighted material

Free Gift

In closing, I want to express my heartfelt gratitude to all readers who have joined us on this enlightening journey into the realm of sexual well-being. Your commitment to self-improvement and personal growth is truly inspiring, and I'm grateful for the opportunity to share valuable insights and strategies with you.

As a token of appreciation for your dedication, I'm thrilled to offer you a complimentary one-month personalized training plan and nutritional guidance to enhance your personal potency. Whether you're aiming to boost physical fitness, increase stamina, or explore new avenues for sexual empowerment, this tailored plan can help you take proactive steps toward achieving your goals.

To claim your free consultation and personalized training plan, simply send an email to frrosato89@gmail.com with a photo of yourself holding the book. I'm excited to collaborate with you and support you on your journey to improved sexual health and vitality.

Thank you once again for your engagement and enthusiasm. Your commitment to personal growth is commendable, and I look forward to assisting you in reaching your full potential.

Best regards,

Francesco Rosato

www.ingramcontent.com/pod-product-compliance
Lightning Source LLC
Chambersburg PA
CBHW070820260726
48660CB00005B/1920